LYN

DRAINAGE

THERAPIES

Cleansing Your Lymphatic System

Support Your Lymphatic System With Therapies That Enhance Detoxification And Strengthen The Immune Response

DR. BRIDGET PROMISE

CHAPTER ONE

Introduction

The human body is a wonder of intricacy, with many different systems coordinating to keep health at its best. The lymphatic system is one of these complex systems that has an important but sometimes overlooked function.

To fully appreciate the lymphatic system's role in preserving general health, one must have a thorough understanding of its operations. We will examine the lymphatic system's complexities in this talk, including its function in detoxification, the essential elements that support its health, and the warning signals of a slow lymphatic system.

Knowledge Of The Lymphatic System

The body's network of organs, veins, and nodes known as the lymphatic system cooperates to move lymph—a colorless fluid that contains white blood cells—around the body.

This system works closely with the circulatory system, enhancing its ability to support the immune system and preserve fluid balance. Nearly every region of the body is covered by the vast network of lymphatic vessels, which run parallel to the blood vessels.

Little bean-shaped structures called lymph nodes serve as filtration points for the lymphatic veins. These nodes are essential for keeping an eye out for dangerous items like viruses and bacteria in the lymph and for triggering the immune system when needed.

The tonsils, thymus, and spleen are also vital lymphatic system components that support general health and immunological function.

The Lymphatic System's Function In Detoxification

Detoxification is one of the lymphatic system's main purposes. Toxins, cellular waste, and other undesirable materials are gathered and transported by the lymphatic fluid as it flows throughout the body to be filtered and removed.

This procedure is essential for preserving a hygienic and salubrious internal milieu, averting the build-up of detrimental agents that may jeopardize cellular performance and general well-being.

Alongside the liver and kidneys, two important organs involved in detoxification, the lymphatic system functions. The lymphatic system assists in moving the byproducts of the liver's processing and neutralization of toxins so they may be eliminated.

Similarly, the lymphatic system assists in eliminating extra fluid and waste products from the kidneys' waste-filtering of the blood. Essentially, the lymphatic system is an essential component of the body's internal cleansing process.

Essential Elements Of A Sound Lymphatic System

To maintain general well-being, the lymphatic system must be kept in good shape. This system works best when a few essential elements are in place, which guarantees that it is effective in detoxifying and supporting the immune system.

1. Hydration: A healthy lymphatic system depends on getting enough water. Since water makes up the majority of lymph, maintaining proper hydration aids in the fluidity of lymphatic fluid and promotes easy passage of the fluid through the capillaries.

2. Nutrition: The lymphatic system is supported in its health by a diet high in nutrients and well-balanced. Foods high in antioxidants, such as fruits and vegetables, support the general health of lymphatic arteries and nodes by reducing inflammation and oxidative stress.

3. Frequent Exercise: Exercise has a major role in boosting lymphatic circulation. The lymphatic system, in contrast to the circulatory system, depends on muscle contraction and movement to transfer lymphatic fluid. Frequent exercise enhances lymphatic flow by supporting this natural

pumping motion, especially those involving rhythmic movements.

4. Deep Breathing methods: Lymphatic drainage may be encouraged by using appropriate breathing methods, such as diaphragmatic breathing. To impact the lymphatic flow and drainage, deep breaths help the diaphragm move more easily.

5. Skin brushing: Exfoliating the skin with a gentle brush that has soft bristles activates the lymphatic system. This method promotes lymphatic circulation, aids in the removal of dead skin

cells, and aids in the skin's ability to expel toxins.

6. Massage and Manual Lymphatic Drainage: Massage treatments, especially those intended for lymphatic drainage, may help to facilitate the flow of lymphatic fluid and lessen congestion. These specialty massages use light, rhythmic strokes to promote the lymphatic system's natural flow.

CHAPTER TWO
Indications Of A Slow
Lymphatic System

Numerous indications and symptoms of a slow lymphatic system may point to the need for care and assistance. It is essential to identify these symptoms to take preventative action and enhance lymphatic function.

1. Edema or persistent swelling: Lymphatic congestion may be the cause of persistent swelling, particularly in the limbs. Fluid buildup from suboptimal lymphatic system function might result in swelling or edema.

2. Recurrent diseases: Recurrent infections or diseases may be brought on by a compromised immune system, which is often linked to a slow lymphatic system. The lymphatic system is essential to the body's protection against infections, and its dysfunction may expose the immune system.

3. Fatigue: Feelings of lethargy and exhaustion may be attributed to lymphatic congestion. Energy levels may be lowered while the body fights to effectively remove pollutants.

4. Digestive Problems: The lymphatic and digestive systems

are intimately related, and obstruction in one may have an impact on the other. Constipation, bloating, and pain in the abdomen are examples of digestive problems that might be a sign of lymphatic problems.

5. Skin Issues: A weakened lymphatic system may be the cause of skin disorders including dryness, acne, or a poor complexion. The removal of waste materials that may have an impact on skin health is facilitated by proper lymphatic drainage.

In summary, the lymphatic system is an essential part of the human body that supports the immune system, aids in detoxification, and promotes general health. Important measures in supporting optimum health include knowing how it works, identifying symptoms of a slow system, and implementing healthy habits.

People may be proactive in ensuring that their lymphatic system functions well by including skin brushing or massage, frequent exercise, good diet, and hydration. Setting this system's health as a top priority may help people achieve a healthy and flourishing sense of well-being.

For general health and well-being to be maintained, the lymphatic system is essential. The lymphatic system, which supports the immune system, removes extra fluid from tissues, and filters dangerous chemicals, has to be properly taken care of to operate at its best. The maintenance and improvement of the health of the lymphatic system may be achieved via a variety of treatments and lifestyle choices.

In this investigation, we examine treatments, dietary plans, and physical exercises that encourage and facilitate the lymphatic system's effective operation.

Treatments That Support The Lymphatic System

Lymphatic Drainage Via Hand

A specific kind of massage called manual lymphatic drainage (MLD) is intended to encourage the body's lymphatic fluid to flow more freely. Professional massage therapists use soft, rhythmic strokes to stimulate lymph flow, which helps eliminate waste, toxins, and extra fluid. Those with lymphedema, a disorder marked by swelling brought on by an accumulation of lymphatic fluid, benefit most from this treatment.

MLD eases stress and, by clearing the lymph nodes of congestion, strengthens the immune system. It helps reduce swelling and promotes the body's natural healing processes, which is why it is often used as part of the recuperation after surgery.

Methods Of Dry Brushing

A simple but powerful technique for promoting lymphatic function is dry brushing. People softly brush certain patterns in their skin using a brush made of natural bristles, usually in the direction of their hearts. This method stimulates the flow of lymphatic fluid, increases blood circulation, and exfoliates the skin.

It is believed that dry brushing stimulates the lymphatic vessels close to the skin's surface, aiding in the removal of toxins and waste. Furthermore, it might enhance the skin's look by diminishing the visibility of cellulite and encouraging a radiant, healthy complexion. Dry brushing is a beneficial self-care practice that may help maintain the lymphatic system's general health.

CHAPTER THREE
Herbal Therapy For A Healthy Lymphatic System

For millennia, traditional medicine has used herbs to promote many body processes, including lymphatic system functioning. Herbal treatments may be used to help detoxification procedures, lower inflammation, and increase lymphatic circulation.

For example, echinacea is well-known for enhancing immunity and supporting the general well-being of the lymphatic system. Another plant that has been historically utilized to enhance circulation and cleanse the lymphatic system is red clover. These herbs may naturally promote lymphatic function when added to drinks or supplements.

Hydration's Effect On The Lymphatic System

Sufficient hydration is necessary for the lymphatic system to operate at its best. Water must be available in sufficient amounts for the lymphatic fluid to carry nutrients and eliminate waste from cells. Hydrated bodies allow the lymphatic vessels to perform their vital roles effectively.

Dehydration may cause the lymphatic system to become lethargic, which impairs the system's capacity to support the immune system and cleanse. As a result, consuming enough water is an essential dietary tactic for promoting lymphatic health. People should make an effort to consume the recommended quantity of water each day, taking into account variables including age, weight, and degree of exercise.

Foods And Supplements That Boost Lymphatic Function

Certain foods and substances may help optimize lymphatic function. Vitamin C-rich citrus fruits have a reputation for boosting immunity and promoting lymphatic health. Leafy greens and cruciferous vegetables, in particular, are rich in phytonutrients and antioxidants that aid in detoxification and lymphatic circulation.

Because of their anti-inflammatory qualities, supplements like omega-3 fatty acids may improve cardiovascular health and reduce inflammation, both of which are beneficial to the lymphatic system. Furthermore, research has been done on the pineapple enzyme bromelain, which may help to enhance circulation and lessen lymphatic congestion.

Exercise And Physical Activity For Lymphatic Health

Maintaining an active lifestyle is essential for the lymphatic system. The lymphatic system, in contrast to the circulatory system, lacks a pump and is dependent on muscular contractions to transport lymphatic fluid throughout the body. Exercises with rhythmic motions, like walking, running, or cycling, may activate and improve the function of the lymphatic system.

Another workout regimen that has been particularly connected to lymphatic health is yoga. Inversions and twists are two yoga positions that encourage the flow of fluid in certain parts of the body, which may aid in lymphatic drainage. Deep breathing techniques, which are popular in yoga, may also improve circulation in general, which is beneficial to the lymphatic system.

Weightlifting and other resistance training exercises help strengthen the lymphatic system. Gaining muscular mass promotes higher metabolic activity, which enhances cardiovascular health generally and lymphatic circulation in particular.

In conclusion, immune system support, detoxification, and general well-being all depend on a functional lymphatic system. Herbal medicines may provide natural help, and therapies like dry brushing and manual lymphatic drainage is efficient ways to encourage lymphatic movement. Nutritional tactics are essential, such as drinking plenty of water and eating foods that stimulate the lymphatic system. For the lymphatic system to work at its best, regular physical activity—including activities that promote lymphatic circulation—is crucial. Including these methods in a holistic wellness regimen may support general health and a robust lymphatic system.

CHAPTER FOUR

Relaxation Techniques To Assist The Lymphatic System

Stress Reduction and Meditation

For millennia, people have used meditation to improve their general well-being, mental clarity, and level of relaxation. According to recent research, stress-reduction methods and meditation may benefit the lymphatic system. Prolonged stress may weaken immunity, cause inflammation, and interfere with the lymphatic system's capacity to effectively eliminate toxins.

People do concentrated breathing and awareness exercises during mindfulness meditation, which encourages a deeply relaxed state of mind. Thus, less stress and less stress hormone production may result from this. The lymphatic system may perform better when stress levels drop, enhancing the immune system and proper fluid drainage.

Even for brief periods, adding meditation to daily routines may have long-term advantages for the lymphatic system. Effective methods for promoting general lymphatic health include gradual muscular relaxation, focused breathing, and guided meditation.

The Effects Of Yoga On Lymphatic Flow

Yoga has become more well-known for its all-encompassing approach to wellness. It is an ancient discipline that incorporates physical postures, breath control, and meditation. Yoga positions and sequences that encourage mobility and drainage are thought to improve the function of the lymphatic system.

It is believed that inverted postures like Legs Up the Wall and

Downward-Facing Dog help lymphatic fluid to flow into the lymph nodes, which aids in detoxifying. Yoga's regular breathing techniques could also activate the lymphatic system, which would help the body expel waste.

Frequent yoga practice enhances general lymphatic circulation in addition to fostering flexibility and strength. Yoga's blend of physical activity, breath awareness, and relaxation may help promote a more robust lymphatic system and overall better health.

External Treatments To Improve The Lymphatic System

The Advantages of Hydrotherapy

Using water in different ways for therapeutic purposes, such as hot and cold compresses, steam baths, or contrast showers, is known as hydrotherapy.

By enhancing cleansing, decreasing inflammation, and increasing circulation, this exercise may benefit the lymphatic system.

Warm water, such as that found in a sauna or warm bath, may help widen lymphatic and blood vessels, which can increase blood flow and make it easier to remove waste. However, cold water—applied as chilly showers or compresses—may narrow blood vessels and reduce swelling, assisting the lymphatic system in its filtration and drainage functions.

It is believed that contrast hydrotherapy, which alternates between hot and cold water, may increase the lymphatic system's pumping function and improve circulation. Including hydrotherapy in a health regimen may help with lymphatic system treatment as well as relaxation.

Compression Clothes To Promote Lymphatic Function

Compression garments are customized clothes designed to put pressure on certain body parts to encourage lymphatic and blood flow. These clothes are often used to treat illnesses including lymphedema, which is characterized by a buildup of lymphatic fluid that causes swelling.

Compression garments can reduce lymphatic channel width by applying external pressure, which makes lymphatic fluid easier to transfer. By preventing the accumulation of extra fluid in the tissues, this compression may encourage effective drainage and lessen edema.

Compression clothing is available in a variety of styles, such as wraps, stockings, and sleeves, and it is designed to fit certain body parts. In addition to being recommended by medical specialists for those with lymphatic diseases, athletes and anyone looking to boost their lymphatic system during extended periods of inactivity or travel may also take them as a preventative measure.

To sum up, integrating external treatments and mind-body activities into one's lifestyle may provide significant assistance to the lymphatic system. The effects of prolonged stress on the lymphatic system are lessened by practicing relaxation methods such as meditation. The exercise, breathing techniques, and meditation included in yoga help improve lymphatic flow in general. By using water therapeutically, hydrotherapy encourages cleansing and circulation. By exerting external pressure, compression garments facilitate effective lymphatic drainage and are especially useful in the treatment of diseases such as lymphedema. Adopting these techniques promotes general health and vigor in addition to a stronger lymphatic system.

Traditional Chinese Medicine (TCM) and acupuncture: For ages, acupuncture has been an essential part of holistic treatment. TCM is the origin of acupuncture. Meridians are pathways that the body's life force, or Qi, is said to flow through in Traditional

Chinese Medicine. To control Qi flow and bring the body back into equilibrium, acupuncture requires carefully placing tiny needles into certain locations along these meridians.

Acupuncture is thought to enhance circulation and energy balance within the lymphatic system, which facilitates waste and toxin elimination via the lymphatic vessels. This procedure may lessen congestion and improve the lymphatic system's general performance. Acupuncture sites specifically addressed for lymphatic support include those in the groin, armpits, and around the neck.

According to research, acupuncture may influence immune cell activity and foster a healthy immunological response via immunomodulatory effects. Acupuncture enhances the immune system's general health by promoting the lymphatic system.

Essential Oils for Lymphatic Support: Renowned for their medicinal qualities, essential oils derived from plants may be useful allies in promoting the lymphatic system. Certain essential oils may aid in promoting lymphatic circulation and are thought to have inherent cleansing qualities.

For example, lemon essential oil is often suggested due to its purifying qualities. In aromatherapy, or when diluted and administered topically, it is believed to assist lymphatic drainage and encourage a normal lymphatic flow. Similarly, it's well known that grapefruit essential oil may help with detoxification procedures and lessen fluid retention.

CHAPTER FIVE

Essential Oil Massage

Lymphatic drainage may also be aided by a little essential oil massage. A calming and supporting massage mix may be made by adding a few drops of essential oils, such as frankincense, juniper berries, or cypress, to a carrier oil, such as coconut or jojoba oil.

Immune System Relationship to Lymphatic Health: It is essential to comprehend how the immune and lymphatic systems interact to fully recognize the importance of maintaining a healthy lymphatic system. The immune system and lymphatic system are closely intertwined, collaborating to protect the body from illnesses and infections.

Important parts of the lymphatic system, the lymph nodes contain immune cells that are essential for identifying and getting rid of infections. Antibodies, immune-related chemicals, and immune cells are efficiently transported throughout the body when the lymphatic system is operating at peak efficiency.

Boosting the Immune Response with Lymphatic Support: The

healthy operation of the lymphatic system is essential for a robust and adaptable immune response. People may strengthen their immune systems generally by implementing habits that promote lymphatic health.

One such technique that encourages lymphatic circulation is regular exercise. The contraction of lymphatic vessels is improved by physical activity, which facilitates the flow of lymphatic fluid. Including exercises such as yoga, swimming, or brisk walking in your regimen may help support immune function by promoting lymphatic health.

Another crucial element in keeping the lymphatic system functioning properly is staying hydrated. Maintaining a healthy fluid balance and preventing lymphatic congestion are two benefits of drinking enough water. Herbal teas may be a refreshing and supporting addition to your daily routine, especially if they include detoxifying qualities.

Including Activities that Promote Lymphatic Health in Your Daily Routine: Including exercises that promote lymphatic health in your daily routine doesn't have to be difficult. Minimal lifestyle changes may have a big impact on lymphatic function promotion.

Using a brush with natural bristles to gently exfoliate the skin is known as "dry brushing." By enhancing blood circulation and lymphatic fluid flow, this technique is said to activate the lymphatic system. Adding soft strokes toward the heart to your daily self-care regimen may be a revitalizing addition to dry brushing before a shower.

A diet rich in fruits, vegetables, and whole foods also promotes general health, which includes lymphatic system health. Antioxidant-rich foods including citrus fruits, berries, and leafy greens may help to boost immunological function and reduce inflammation.

Summary

Alternative treatments provide beneficial options for those who want to develop and maintain their lymphatic system. By encouraging proper lymphatic function, acupuncture, traditional Chinese medicine, and essential oils may supplement traditional medical procedures.

Comprehending the relationship between the immune system and the lymphatic system emphasizes how crucial it is to maintain a healthy lymphatic system for general health. People may actively enhance their immune response and general health by implementing easy habits like exercising, drinking enough water, and using a dry brush.

Before implementing alternative treatments, like with any health-related activity, it is recommended to speak with healthcare specialists, particularly for those who already have medical concerns. A thorough and individualized strategy for lymphatic health and immune support might benefit from a holistic approach that incorporates traditional and alternative medicine.

Printed in Great Britain
by Amazon

38761543R10030